HAIRSTYLIST 101

Tips, Tricks, Tools & Techniques That
Turn Beginners Into Pros

RAYMOND NEGRON

CONTENTS

INTRODUCTION

Hairstylist 101

I've always had a fascination with hair, from the time I was a kid, doing my cousin's and sister's hair and playing with my favorite toy Barbie. She had black, knee-length hair and I enjoyed giving her as many hairstyles as I could. I would sit there alone and marvel at the creations I came up with. Hairstyling was an escape for me, it was something I was naturally good at. My grandma always knew I was destined for this. She would always say, "You're going to grow up to be a great hairstylist one day." Little did she know I would grow up to be an author too.

I remember like it was yesterday when my parents gave me my first pair of haircutting shears.

It was the end of summer '99, and after I'd decided to pursue a career in the beauty industry. I enrolled myself as a part-time student while still completing a full college term schedule. Beauty school was very different from what I pictured it to be. I never thought there were so many requirements needed to become a licensed cosmetologist. You see, beauty school is not just where you learn the trendiest techniques or where you discover what kind of stylist you want to be. Along with learning about hair, skin, and nails, you learn about the anatomy of the head, including bones and structures. These are things I didn't know I needed to know but actually turned out to be pretty interesting.

Within my first week, I realized I didn't know how to hold my shears properly. Ever since I started practicing cutting hair in my teens, I had always used my middle finger in place of where the ring finger belonged. When my teacher saw this she chuckled and gently grabbed my hand. She looked at me and said, "let's work on that *finger positioning shall we*". She helped to guide me and moved my fingers to the correct position. For the first time, I realized I was now holding my shears like a professional. It was like a light bulb went off. I couldn't have known how much more comfortable it would feel to position my fingers where they needed to be instead of guessing how to hold my shears. From that moment on, I felt my confidence soar. I knew I would be destined to become a great hairstylist.

Over the last two decades, I became a well-rounded hairstylist specializing in styling, cutting, coloring and hair installations. Although I took classes and workshops, a lot of what I learned was from trial and error. It also took many years to figure out the blueprints of effective time management, customer service, and overall salon etiquette. This book will fast-forward your learning and put into perspective things I wish I had known before I entered this business. I will share with you some of my favorite tools and products and how to use them to "WOW" your clients. We will delve into coloring terminology, giving you clear and concise formulas for hair color and a simplified break down of various coloring techniques.

After reading Hairstylist 101, you will be ready to take control of your career. Not only will you know how to master the techniques enclosed, but you will learn the foundation of great customer service. You will learn how to be confident, professional, and responsible. You will be able to give a client a thorough consultation and how to command the right price for your expertise.

This book is organized into four parts: techniques and tools for cutting hair, techniques for coloring hair, tools and products, and the business of hairstyling. I'll reveal vital information to master these techniques and tools and will help you think outside the box by encouraging you to work from your gut, think with your mind, and create from your heart.

For additional information and resource material, I welcome you to visit my site at www.hairstylist101.com.

Section 1:

All Things Cutting

CHAPTER 1

The Consultation

The initial consultation is by far the most crucial part of the communication between you and your client. This is where you will discover what they like and don't like, what they want and don't want, and where you will be given the opportunity to provide your professional recommendations. It's imperative to remain focused when discussing different ideas and to ensure you understand your client's hair history. Remember to stay focused on the client. Eye contact and a true dialogue go far; they impart trust and mutual respect, which are both vital before, during and after a hair appointment.

If performing a color service, you must discuss in detail what other color services the client has had in the past. You will need to understand your client's hair history to determine if they have had any chemical services that would affect the process', or to understand other reasons why it may not be a good idea to perform the work being requested. If what's being asked is not a good idea, you must remember to educate your client and suggest a better alternative. Trust me, your client will appreciate it if you give them several options to choose from. There will be times where you will get a client who insists you do something that you feel is not recommended and may compromise the hair's overall integrity. When this happens, it is my suggestion that you communicate that you cannot guarantee the results they are looking for. Remember that it's your professional credibility at stake. It's important to be upfront and honest with the client to ensure the right expectations are set.

When consulting about a drastic haircut of eight inches or longer, encourage the client to donate their hair. There are so many organizations that take hair donations that are at least eight inches and make wigs for cancer patients. Remind them of the gratification they'll feel knowing that their hair has helped to put a smile on someone's face.

During a consultation, it's important that you understand how long a service will take in order to accommodate them into your schedule. Remember, this consultation helps with the flow of the appointment and to control your overall day. Being on schedule makes you look professional and ensures trust between you and the client. By now, your client should feel comfortable with you, and you can proceed to either pre-cutting the hair or go right into shampooing.

In the next chapter will guide you through different shampoo options, and whether or not you will need to use a separate conditioner as well.

CHAPTER 2

Shampoo and Conditioning

Every great hairstyle begins with choosing the proper shampoo and conditioner for the type of hair your client has and the look they are trying to achieve. This is often the client's favorite part of the service. It can be so relaxing to get your hair washed and your scalp massaged before a service. Although it can be relaxing, remember it's important to constantly communicate with your client, ensuring that they are comfortable with the pressure of your massage and that the temperature of the water is okay. Everyone is different, so you may get special requests like two shampoos or the use of a special product prescribed by their dermatologist. Regardless, the key is to make the shampooing process a pleasant experience.

There are many different types of hair, to match this there are also many different types of shampoos and conditioners for each hair. For example, you shouldn't use shampoo for dry and damaged hair on fine hair, and shampoo for oily hair should not be used on colored hair. Using the appropriate shampoo and conditioner for the hair type will give you optimum results. If you're working on hair that's prone to being greasy and you use shampoo with moisture, it will make it more lifeless, as greasy hair lacks volume and bounce.

Below, I have categorized shampoos from one to five, from the least amount of moisture to the most, covering each hair type.

Number One: Shampoo for Oily Hair. When someone has oily hair, it means natural oils develop in their scalp, and they need more cleansing to soak up the oils. Shampoos that say "amplify" or "dry shampoo" are great for greasy, oily hair. Usually, this hair type does not need much conditioner. If it is needed, you should only use a dime or nickel-sized amount, conditioning from mid-shaft down to the tips of the hair.

Number Two: Shampoo for Normal Hair. Normalizing shampoos are probably the most popular type of shampoos.

They are made with just the right amount of moisture needed to hydrate the follicles, and these shampoos don't leave the hair greasy after a wash. This choice of shampoo is perfect for children, men, virgin hair, and provide an overall cleansing of the scalp without removing too much of the moisture. Here's a tip: unless normal hair is way below shoulder-length or prone to tangling, I only suggest using conditioner from the mid-shaft down. That said, if it isn't needed, conditioner can be skipped altogether.

Number Three: Shampoo for Color-treated Hair. Color-treated shampoos and conditioners are unsurprisingly formulated specifically for color-treated hair. Most are made without sulfates and other ingredients to reduce stripping and removal of color pigment. Their formulas are specially made to protect color-treated strands. Some even have color pigments in them to maintain your shade while still providing a cleansing. Depending on the color service that's been done, such as hair lightening, scalp bleach, or high-lift highlights, conditioner should be used to further protect and moisturizes the delicate tresses.

Number Four: Shampoo for Keratin-treatment-treated Hair. Shampoos and conditioners created for chemical keratin treatments are crucial in maintaining the effects of the keratin treatment. These formulas are also made without sulfates or other harsh chemicals that loosen the keratin put in by the service. Just because most of them don't lather with tons of suds does not mean you don't get a good wash. Sulfates give the suds, and people mistakenly believe that the more they're able to create a lather, the cleaner the hair. Wrong! Sulfates are infamous for stripping hair, and the last thing you want is straw or hay-like hair! Keratin clients should only be given this type of shampoo, even if they have color treatments as well.

Number Five: Shampoo for Dry or Damaged Hair. Shampoos and conditioners for dry and damaged hair are the most moisturizing and the heaviest. They provide a gentle cleaning, leave the hair super soft and help to ensure that the hair maintains the moisture it needs. This shampoo and conditioner duo are a must for coarse or curly hair that barely gets moisture. This can help preserve the integrity of the hair. Another tip, if the shampoo and conditioner are too heavy, you can use a normalizing shampoo to reduce the moisture. Dry and damaged hair types almost always need conditioner. Some may need it from the roots down, and others may just need conditioning from the mid-shaft down.

There are also shampoos and conditioners like Head & Shoulders, Neutrogena T-Gel, and Selsun Blue. These shampoos and conditioners are made for people with dandruff or need medicated shampoos for certain seasonal dandruff or psoriasis. In some cases, the client may need a dermatologist recommended special shampoo. Irritation or dandruff should not be overlooked on a client.

With some questioning and research, you can find an appropriate shampoo and conditioner for their hair type. What you need to look for in shampoo and conditioner is one that will act as and will support the base for the overall style. A proper shampoo will clean the hair, and the right conditioner will detangle it effectively.

Now that we have covered the different types of shampoo and conditioners, it's time for us to go to the salon chair to start detangling the now clean and wet hair. We'll then section for the cut or style we are looking to create.

In the next chapter, we will discuss which combs work best for each hair type.

CHAPTER 3

Combs

Combs come in many shapes and sizes. There are fine-tooth combs, wide-tooth combs, short combs, and long combs. There are pin combs and pick combs. Different combs are designed for different hair textures. For instance, you want to use a pick comb for detangling curly hair. Picks have a gentle way of combing through curly hair and gently detangling very long hair. The wider the teeth on the comb, the easier it is to detangle hair. When the teeth are close together, you get clean, tight tensions by creating uniform shape and movement. It's best to use a straight comb for parting and cutting.

Cutting combs are crucial, they help with carving out sections to cut and create with them. Pintail combs are a half comb, with a tapered thin handle. Some pintail combs have a metal tip, designed for weaving strands for highlighting and color effects. Pintail combs are also great for teasing and detailing the hair. The thin handle makes hairstyling and highlighting a breeze. They also help with fluffing and squeezing out any height that may be needed when doing hair for weddings or for doing styles which require volume and or balanced height.

I'm very particular with combs. I prefer to cut with a styling comb that is at least eight inches long and has fine teeth on one half and wider teeth on the other. I can grab thick hair with a breeze and lay a great cutting foundation with these combs. I prefer combs that are durable and sturdy. When I find a comb I really like, I guard it with my life and take great care of it. Combs are just as important as your shears.

In the next chapter, we will discuss the importance of sectioning and clips along with their different types and uses.

CHAPTER 4

Sectioning and Clips

Sectioning is the art of separating the hair you are working with from the hair you are not working with. It is crucial in all aspects of hair artistry. When sectioning hair, you can choose to make straight parts, diagonal parts, or zigzag parts. Hair sectioning is used in cutting, coloring, highlighting, chemical work, and styling. For example, sectioning for a haircut allows you to work in a designated area, creating a guideline for the sections that will follow.

Sectioning in hair color keeps the process neat and concise. Using different patterns of sectioning for highlighting hair make the effects of highlighting a true art. Sectioning sets the foundation of every style, haircut, and chemical procedure. Sectioning is especially crucial with thick hair. You need to section thick hair away from other sections when cutting. Also, thick hair should be sectioned several times during blow dries. I love to section my parts diagonally when I blow dry. Using the right clips can make a huge difference when sectioning as well.

Duck bill clips are 3-to 4-inch aluminum clips that have a curve to them with multiple uses. For instance, they are excellent for holding a thermal curl until it cools. The curve of a duck bill clip helps it easily stay in place close to the head. Bigger plastic clips are typical for cutting and coloring. Some have an extra jagged claw to grab thicker hair tightly. Also made with a curve, they glide and let you place your sections neatly and securely. Clips can also be small and claw-like, to sweep bangs out of the way or to drag a few strands together. Overall, sections and clips are the perfect marriage; when choosing the right one they complement each other and make your job much easier.

In the next chapter, we will talk about shears and scissors and how to choose the right pair.

CHAPTER 5

Shears

Usually, when we think of shears, we think of basic scissors. They're a tool to cut and that's it. However, we don't give enough credit to haircutting shears. Shears are like the pen to the poet. Sure, you need the canvas, but the right tool will make you comfortable enough to execute your vision.

There are many different models of shears to choose from, including shears for left-handed stylists. Shears are ergonomically designed to not only be comfortable in their finger positioning but in the length of the blade. When cutting with shorter shears, you will use more frequent strokes, while a longer-blade shear will cut most sections in one shot. It all boils down to control and how you like the comfort and slice of the shear. Different models of shears have varying details, they come in different sizes, shapes, materials, and coloring. Japanese and German blades offer the best in professional steel shears. My preference is a long-blade shear. My favorite pair is seven inches long, with a very sharp blade.

Yet I cannot stress enough that blades are delicate. If you drop your shears and they bang on the ground, they will nick the blade. Only an experienced shear-sharpener can fix these nicks, and good sharpeners are hard to find.

Shears can range from $25 to $500, and some go for even more than that. When first starting out in the beauty industry, find yourself a nice basic set of shears, get used to them and understand how to take care of them. As you get more experienced you can start to purchase more expensive pairs to build up your arsenal of shears. Remember you can always upgrade to a better-quality steel shear at any time. Eventually, you'll create your team of shears and other tools that make the art of haircutting wonderful.

So far we have covered the consultation, washing, combs, sectioning, clips, and shears. Let's move forward and dive into the fun part.

In the next chapter, you are going to want to start cutting right away. I will share a pattern cutting description and a step-by-step way to do my signature shaggy layered cut.

CHAPTER 6

Pattern Cutting

When cutting hair, it is important to assess the hair and to decide what pattern you will use to create their desired look. Following a pattern will make sure you follow the appropriate steps to ensure you get the right look every time. For instance, this is my pattern for cutting a long-layered haircut.

First, I begin by sectioning the hair and establishing the length. I then move to the front of the hair and decide if we'll use a middle part, a side part, or bangs as a starting point. At this point, if we have decided to cut the bangs, I do. If we have agreed on a middle or a side part, I will take a tiny section from both partings and cut out a guideline. Depending on what the starting layer will be, I usually use various points on the face for reference—the bridge of the nose, the tip of the nose, the lips, the chin, or below the chin.

At this point, once I've decided on the starting layer, I face-frame from the starting guideline and cut using the slither technique. The slithering technique is achieved with a very sharp blade and a steady hand motion. I position my shear at the guideline and slither down to the length. For example, if the client wants short, shaggy layers with no bangs, I would cut the starting point at the bridge of the nose, then face-frame evenly on both sides. The same pattern applies if cutting on a side part; just keep in mind if you position it back in the middle, it will be uneven. Side part cuts should only be used on someone who always wears their hair to the side.

Now that I've done the length and the face-frame, I grab a one-inch Mohawk section from the front of the hairline to the crown right before it rounds to the back of the head. This one-inch section will be the shortest layer and will serve as the guideline for blending into the length. After I have cut my guideline, I divide it in half and begin to work on one side of the head. Taking one-inch pie sections, I carefully cut down to the length. If I'm working on the left side of the head first, I make a cut then go to the same spot on the right side and do the same cut. This ensures balance and keeps the layering consistent. I then work beside that section, cut and repeat it on the other side of the head. I continue this process until I reach the middle of the back part of the head.

Using this pattern for a shaggy haircut has never failed me. Whether doing a short shag or a long one, this technique ensures even and consistent results. Once you become more experienced, you will start to create your own guidelines, steps and signature patterns.

In the next chapter, we get creative and experience what I call custom cutting. Custom cutting is used to create specific shapes for what the client is looking for.

CHAPTER 7

Custom cutting

Custom cutting is the art of making a haircut work on different people. Not everyone has the same shape head, nor does the same style of hair flatter every client. Everyone is unique. Custom cutting individualizes a hairstyle for someone. There are times in the art of hairstyling that you must modify, or even create movement or disappearance in the shaping of the hair. Some of the greatest custom cutting shapes include mohawks, textured lobs (longer version of a bob), undercut wedges, bangs, and side-swept bangs/layers. People who are gifted with an exuberant amount of hair are also excellent opportunities for a custom cut.

I have a client I've been styling for the last five years who has an amazing head of course, thick hair. My favorite texture to shape and style. When I first started doing her hair, she stressed that she loved the length of her hair and wouldn't mind layering it, but she needed its thickness considerably reduced. Her hair was just about waist length, I decided we would cut about three inches from the length and reduce the bulk of hair with a thinning/texturizing shear. Reducing the thickness in hair could be a whole other chapter. I can go on and on about different ways to reduce thickness, whether at the root or mid-shaft or just the tips. Some more details on thinning out hair are given in chapter 9. When working on this client, I decreased her hair density by about 35%, especially in the areas where heaviness remains, such as the back crown, occipital area, and the nape area.

Another example of a custom cut is a gentleman whose hair I've cut for the past eight years. He has an undercut and likes to get his center, longer hair texturized from the mid-shaft down, giving the ends a wispier texture.

As a hairstylist remember that you are also an artist, custom cutting allows you to give someone a more personalized look. By the end of your consultation with the client and considering the client expectations you should know whether you will use a pattern cut or a customized cut. There is no right or wrong way to cut just listen to what your client is asking for and it will come to you. Talk through your final recommendations for the cut and enjoy the ride as you give the client a brand-new look.

Cutting the hair can also be done with a razor. In the next chapter, we will go through my uses for the razor. Specifically when, where, and how to use it.

CHAPTER 8

Using a Razor

To achieve funky cut lines in a haircut or a deconstructed shape like those used in custom cutting, having different tools and knowing how and when to use them is key. Using a razor alone for a haircut can be tricky. Razors are sharp and the tension used on the hair will change the effect they give. Heavy tension will create a bulky, feathered tip, while a light tension stroke can create a more controlled, flowy, feathered look.

Razors are excellent for side-swept bangs, softening a blunt line, and thinning out very thick hair. They are best used, in my opinion, after a scissor cut to detail any hard lines. I love to use a razor after the blow-dry to soften the edges of a haircut. I rake the hair between my fingers and graze the razor along my palm, skimming the last two inches of hair or less. This gives softer ends within a more structured cut.

There are also electric hot razors. These razors vibrate and heat up the blade. When cutting with it, the heat seals the cuticle and minimizes frizz on curly hair. It works particularly well with hair extensions and thick, one-length hair, giving soft, textured ends. Both handle razors and electric razors use the same replacement blades. Haircutting blades usually come in a pack and make replacing a fresh one simple. You pull out a new blade, replace the old one, and continue cutting.

You can even get temporary razors. These are razors built into a disposable handle so you can throw them away after they have become dull. Lastly, razors are great for custom cutting. Using different tensions and strokes can create personalized looks. While I think it's best to tread slowly, take advantage of willing clients and friends who would let you experiment. This is where creativity will take the lead and you'll be having fun at work in no time.

Thinning and texturizing hair is a skill that takes practice. In the next chapter, I will explain the thinning shear and a breakdown of how I like to use it on my clients.

CHAPTER 9

Thinning Shears

Thinning shears are scissors with a blade on one side and a comb blade on the other. The purpose of this shear is to decrease the density in the hair. Using this tool is great for removing bulk evenly or when more controlled thinning is desired. The bigger the teeth on the comb blade, the more density is removed. The finer the comb blade, the lighter the effect will be.

Not every hair texture needs thinning or reducing. However, it can make a big difference in creating balance. For example, let's say you have a client who wants to have their bangs cut and wants a softer look. Pick up the blunt bangs up with the comb in a 90-degree angle and chip into the last inch of the bangs with a series of steady, repeated strokes. Continue to detail until you get the desired look. The end result will give softer-looking bangs that are very flattering.

Using the shears in a parallel motion will make the cut more discreet, while perpendicular use will make the cut more obvious through the strands. When thinning out very thick heads of hair, I will use the thinning shear in a perpendicular motion in a strategic pattern. This decreases weight considerably and gives the illusion of a much more balanced head of hair.

There is an art to creating good growth outlines with these shears. Since bigger teeth remove larger chunks, they can give the illusion of holes if not cut right. Using these shears parallel or diagonally can soften the cuts and hide them effectively under the layers on top of them.

You can thin out hair wet or dry. I usually decide when I'll thin hair based on the length or overall look. I prefer to thin out long hair after the blow dry. It makes removing bulk easier and the hair slides out after a good brushing. Especially on long or thick hair, remember to thin and brush out the hair in sections. Thinning out the entire head without brushing it out in small increments will result in a tangled mess. All the loose hair will clump like a reverse tease and make it impossible to brush.

The final chapter in this section is dedicated to hair clippers. In this chapter we'll discuss using a pattern or custom undercutting, these tools in conjunction with shears make drastic and effective shapes.

CHAPTER 10

Clippers, Edgers, and Detailers

Hair clippers are essential when a buzzed, faded, or undercut look is desired. Clippers have attachment guards to regulate different lengths between one inch and 1/16 inch. Clippers can be used for skin-tight effects or when even consistency is needed. They either have plastic, measured attachments or actual clipper blade attachments. The one you choose is merely a matter of preference.

Edgers and detailers provide the tightest, closest cut you can get. They are used to finish sideburns, even out hairlines, or even to carve out parts and to stencil effects in hair. Clippers quickly remove hair evenly, so it's best to tread lightly and understand how the lengths work. You don't want to go too short. Also, remember that lighter hair looks much shorter than dark hair when using clippers, so make sure you know the different sizes to recommend the best setting for your clients look.

There are cordless models, which makes getting around the head a breeze, but I find using clippers and edgers with power cords more effective for me. This keeps the speed and power consistent and alleviates having to make sure you charge your buzzers.

Keeping them clean and oiled will prolong the life of their blades and will ensure to keep them sanitary after every use. After a while, you'll notice the blades become dull and you'll need a new blade attachment. Luckily, all you may need is a replacement blade. If kept in great shape and wrapped properly at the end of a cut, the clipper itself will have a long life. However, if you mistakenly drop them, you can damage vital parts inside. Treat clippers gently and remember to wrap the cord loosely around it when done. If wound too tight, it can pull on the power cord and create a shortage. A mistake you want to avoid

That concludes all things cutting, from the consultation to using the right shears and tools used to cut. In the next section, we'll discuss hair coloring. The first chapter of this part will be the hair-coloring-specific version of the consult: the patch test.

Section 2:

All Things Color

CHAPTER 11

A Patch Test

Like a consultation, a patch test is important, especially when working on someone for the first time. In fact, it is the most important part of a color consultation. A patch test can save you a great deal if you have any doubts whatsoever. The test can let you know if the client can receive scalp procedures, if they are allergic to any hair colors or dyes, or if the ammonia or peroxide will be abrasive on the client's sensitive skin. You want your client to trust that you have their best interests at heart and to know that you put their safety first.

A patch test will also test how long a process will take. When hair is virgin of chemicals and color, it makes lifting and using chemicals splendid. Most virgin hair processes are fast and gentle. If a person has staining from previous metallic hair dyes or dark dyes, extracting from the hair can take a long time. It can lift unevenly or in some cases it can compromise the hair's integrity. The same goes for chemical straighteners, body waves, and perms. A patch test could derail your whole idea but in a good way. It could save you from doing something totally disastrous. Fixing a disaster could affect your scheduling and any other clients you may have that day.

Also, a patch test will determine if the service will be a simple color correction or a more complex service that will need you to devote a few hours to. If after the test it turns out the process will be more complex, be ready to explain to your client any changes in the pricing since it may be more than they were wanting to spend. When performing a color correction the client should always sign a waiver. The waiver is a terms and conditions agreement both parties agree to. For example, a waiver may include the procedure, time, price and a plan B if necessary. When a person wants you to guarantee results, they expect to get what they pay for. Remember to be open, honest and state the facts so you do not put your reputation at risk.

You should not guess or overpromise. You will get yourself in a bind if you assume, so always do a patch test. In some instances, coloring will take more than one visit, remember to explain the process in detail.

With new hair products launching all the time and new techniques being utilized, it is important you and the client are on the same page, so educate them on their terminology versus your professional terminology. Clients tend to appreciate this so don't hesitate in making the communication clear to ensure they understand the correct terms used in hair coloring. It will speed things along in future sessions.

In the next chapter, we will break down the color wheel, along with the different levels and the different tones. Once you learn the color wheel, levels, and tones, you will never look at hair color the same. You will constantly refer back to it and will become an amazing colorist.

CHAPTER 12

The Color Wheel – Levels & Tones

The color wheel is the greatest tool in hair color. I remember when my instructor explained the laws of color. He used a blank white wall as an example and he said if you paint a stripe of blue and go over the same stripe with red and go over the same stripe with yellow, you get brown. As funny as the analogy was, I pictured it perfectly in my brain and instantly became fascinated with laws of color, whether neutralizing or targeting an underlying pigment.

The color wheel is your valuable tool. The laws of color will never change. The color wheel is divided as the three primaries: red, yellow, and blue, and secondary colors which are colors made from two of the primary colors. Red and yellow make orange, yellow and blue make green, and blue and red make violet. Tertiary colors are colors made with primary and secondary colors. For example, if you have brassy, yellow-orange hair and want to neutralize, you would use a green-blue base. If your hair is pure yellow or golden, you would use a violet base. To neutralize, all three primary colors must be present.

Tones are the color hue that exists in each level. Golden and warm are examples of tones. They appear lighter and more vibrant. Warm red tones also look lighter for their reflective tones. Ash and cool tend to look darker and more natural. Whether wanting to cancel a tone or intensify the tone, the color wheel is your reference for target results.

When analyzing a client's hair, we want to locate its level and underlying pigment. Levels are numbers to describe dark to light, blue-black being level 1 and white being level 11. The following is a chart explaining the law of color and the underlying pigment found in each of the hair colors.

Levels 1-11

- 11 white—platinum, gray, silver and salt-and-pepper strands: ash cool
- 10 pale blondes—pale yellow, vanilla: ash cool
- 9 blonde—yellow, beige, champagne: cool-neutral
- 8 medium blonde—yellow, golden, sandy neutral-warm but no red exists
- 7 dark blonde—yellow-orange, warm, honey, warm gold present
- 6 light brown—orange, copper, bronze, chestnut, warm gold-orange
- 5 medium brown—red orange, fiery, Auburn, crimson
- 4 dark brown—red undertones, dark auburn, ruby, scarlet, red most present
- 3 darkest brown—deep red and violet undertones, eggplant, and mahogany
- 2 soft black—neutral, warm undertone, only visible if you put up to the light
- 1 blue-black—ash base underlying pigment, barely visible, cool deep blue base

CHAPTER 13

Brassy vs. Mousy

These are the terms most people get confused about when determining what they want to convey regarding what they don't like about their hair. Clients will say things like, "My hair is *brassy*," or "My hair is *orange*." This means there is a very warm, brassy tone whether from using hair color to lighten dark hair or if the color has oxidized through washing it has created a brassy orange or gold tone. In order to avoid a brassy result, a skilled colorist must pre-lighten past brassy tones before a toner gets applied. You must neutralize warmth using an appropriate ash-toned color.

Three examples of those most prone to dealing with brassy hair are single-process users attempting to go light, double-process users who lighten and then high-light with lightener, and brunettes that use colors that are too warm.

I had a client who would single-process her hair at home and would say, "My hair is so *brassy*". I asked her what she used, and she replied, "Light golden brown". Now, if you're a colorist, you understand that a natural level 3 to 4 dark brown attempting to go lighter using a golden-toned base to look like the model on the box, will not give the results they desired. She was intensifying the warmth by adding the golden-tone brown color. Natural dark hair has a deep red tone that can arise when attempting to lighten, and red exists in dark hair even if you can't tell. It's what keeps brunettes rich-looking. Had she used an ash brown instead of the golden brown, she would have gotten a neutral brown tone.

Now mousy, ashy, and drab are all words to describe a tone in the hair. Mousy hair can come in many shades. You can be a mousy blonde, you can be a mousy red, you can even be a mousy brunette. Whether gray hair is making your hair appear mousy or your color has no shine or oomph to it, having mousy hair can actually be a good thing as it can be great for glazes, demi-permanent shades, the different blending of highlights, and going blonder since the hair isn't brassy. Ash is a blue, green or violet base color used to neutralize red, orange and yellow toned hair. Not neutralizing properly can leave you under toned or over toned, where you will see green, blue, or violet. Nowadays, ashy pastel colors are desired, so over toning is used to intensify these colors. Most of these ashy pastels are achieved either on natural gray, white, or pre-lightened hair. In order to see these tones, remember to first remove the pigment on the dark hair.

Here's a great formula to use on a natural level 5 and under who wants to be Nordic, icy blonde. First, you must pre-lighten the hair shaft an inch off the root and an inch from the ends and process until yellow. Depending on the volume strength, this can take up to 40 minutes. The reason you want to avoid the roots and ends is that the middle part of the hair shaft takes the longest to lighten. Applying pre-lightener to the roots will process quickly due to body heat, and because hair ends are porous, they can lighten fast as well.

Next, apply on the roots and ends and continue to process until the color is an even, pale yellow—not white. The hair is now ready for violet-toned ash; these toners work between 10 and 20 minutes, tops. The violet in the ash will neutralize the pale yellow and will leave you with a beautiful, natural light blonde look. If the hair is lightened past pale yellow until it looks white, the same violet ash toner would appear lilac-like. It would be considered over-toned unless you desired that effect.

Drab hair lacks shine and could be a wrong color choice that doesn't suit someone. Or the color isn't flattering because of their skin and eye color. A client may have the perfect skin to be a lustrous redhead or a sultry brown but prefers colors that wash them out without being willing to change to something that might complement them better. While it's best for a client to discuss with a professional what colors would suit them, the wearer must be comfortable with their choice. If a client insists on a color that doesn't suit them, I believe you should grant their wishes. Just stress to them that your most complimented clients are the ones who take your recommendations as a professional.

While this chapter gives a great formula to avoid brassy or mousy results, the next chapter will explain in detail hair color uses and how to mix with the proper developer for different effects.

CHAPTER 14

Hair Color and Developers

When it comes to hair color, there is a rainbow of shades and techniques involved. There are so many factors to consider. Are we covering gray? Are we making the hair brighter? Are we making it darker? Are we highlighting/lowlighting?

Each technique has its place when it comes to the person wearing the color. There is also terminology to explain what a person might want or need. For example, a single-process. The single-process is when you are applying color to all the hair, creating full-strand coverage at once. A single-process is usually used to cover gray, matching hair color, create a new base, or to tone the hair. The normal amount of time for a session is usually 30 to 45 minutes, the longer end if you have a high-lift blonde and or have stubborn, resistant gray hair. It is important when doing gray coverage to mix the color right before applying it and to time it for no more than 45 minutes, for a single-process formula mix can't work any further. Single processes can also be used to deepen and/or tone the hair color within 10 to 20 minutes.

Hair color is divided into two parts. The color portion determines the level and tone, and the developer portion decides if you are toning, covering gray, or high-lifting. Developers have ranges including 10-, 20-, 30-, and 40-volume. 10-volume gives tone or a very slight lift, while 20-volume gives maximum gray coverage and/or two levels of lift. 30-volume gives three levels of lift and 40-volume gives four levels of lift. While I've seen developers go as high as 80-volume promoting very high lifts, after 50-volume I draw the line. Anything after that is either too fast or too complicated to guarantee results.

While I always recommend visiting a salon professional to create foolproof methods and formulas, there are drug store hair color products available for clients to use if they choose.

If they mention this, just relay that you are not responsible for the results and if they do come to you to fix something, it will be considered a color correction. Remember once again to present the waiver if needed.

This concludes the chapter on hair color and developer. In the next chapter, we will focus on another important hair color agent, the lightener. Lightner gets activated by developers and when done right can transform even the darkest head of hair.

CHAPTER 15

Hair Lightening, Decolorizing, Bleach

There would not be a world of possibilities in hair color if hair lightener did not exist. It is responsible for some of the most coveted locks, from Marilyn Monroe's signature blonde to the highlighted effects and the rainbow hair we see around us every day. Even the softest brown tones need decolorizing to reduce warmth and red. Every great colorist uses hair lighteners to make magic.

Hair lightener is known to clients as "*bleach*" when mixed with the developer it creates a product that lifts out both natural and artificial pigment in the hair. Hair color and developers can lift and tone up to four levels on virgin hair as discussed in the last chapter, where lightener can lift up to nine levels. This process can also be referred to as decolorizing, especially when color correction is needed.

Hair lightening is essential in almost all color corrections, it lifts out old artificial pigments and balances levels in the hair color. Hair lightener works on timing. Where you apply product first will be the lightest. Depending on the desired effect, you must work strategically and quickly. Using lower developers can slow down the process where more control is needed, and higher developers can speed up an area. If used incorrectly lighteners can also lead to a compromise in the hair's integrity. You must diagnose the head of hair and discuss honestly if they can get the color service done.

For example, let's say you have a client growing out dyed black hair who wants to become blonde. It's a common request at a salon and it is our duty as hair professionals to educate our clients and weigh their options. In this case, I would explain the process and how each stage affects the hair and what to expect. Also, before any decolorizing is completed, the hair would need a few color extractor services, along with deep conditioning in between. **Do not** apply hair lightener on to freshly washed scalp. It will be abrasive, painful and the client will feel like fire at the scalp. The client should not wash their hair for at least 24-48 hours when scalp lightening is to be done

There have been new product advancements in hair science that you can add to your hair lighteners and hair color that can actually protect your hair. These products when used in your formula, can help to keep the hair bond strong while lightening. Brands like *Olaplex, b3 Brazilian Bond Builder, BOND Ultim8* and *PH Bonder by Redken* are highly recommended. Also, artificial hair color extractors can be used to remove layers of built up dyes leaving less work in the decolorization process. Color extractors are a liquid product that gently removes and lighten any direct dyes and dark patches from previous dye jobs. *Pravana* artificial haircolor extractor is marvelous, makes breaking through dark dyed bases a breeze while still keeping it in great condition. It is definitely worth performing color extractors before attempting to go really light on a client.

Another common request is attempting to remove artificial red tones in the hair. Hair lightener will be used to lift past the red tone and prepare for a neutral or ash base. Hair lightener used on virgin dark hair can be lifted too many different levels, which makes for easy creating on a clean canvas. It is much easier to create a magnitude of color options on unprocessed hair. Again, this is where performing a patch test on a strand will save you time and help you figure out what to expect from the process.

It is time to move on to techniques in hair coloring. In the next chapter, we will explain the double process and how and when its needed.

CHAPTER 16

Double process

A double process is exactly what it sounds like. Whether it's highlights following a single process or highlighting and tone, a double process always involves two processes. Most high-fashion hair colors will receive a double process. For example, when wanting to be a very light wheat color on shades darker than a level 7 dark blonde, you must decolorize first to a pale yellow, then tone to the desired tone. Any color surpassing four levels must be decolorized to receive proper tone, otherwise, unwanted warmth will exist.

Most red or warm colors can be achieved with high-lift colors and higher volumes, but if you are single-processed dark, you must first decolorize, then tone. Color cannot lift color. The discussion in chapter 12 on the color wheel explains this in an almost foolproof way. Only people with naturally light hair or a full head of gray can experience a double-process like result from a single process because of the natural light or gray pigment.

Ultimately, double processes work hand-in-hand to create the most drastic results and promote guaranteed lifting capabilities and tones to spare. However, double processes are also time-consuming, and repeated washing and timing may take place. Prepare your client to be at the salon for a few hours, remember to ask if they will also be getting a haircut and styling as well.

Colorists may take another client while another one is waiting, juggling between the two processes. This way of working is effective because a colorist can apply another base color or put in some highlights for one client while timing the other for 30 or 45 minutes. However, if a client needs a color correction, balancing another client can be tricky.

The following section describes highlights and low lights and the various ways of utilizing these techniques in hair coloring.

CHAPTER 17

Highlights and Lowlights

The art of highlighting and lowlighting is best described as the art of accentuating lines and movement in the hair. Highlighting and lowlighting can be very flattering. If a client wants to add pop to a single area or over their whole head, highlighting is definitely the way to go. You can create drastic highlights with hair lightener and higher volume, or you can highlight with hair color and high volume, or intentionally lowering the volume, depending on the intensity.

Lowlights are the opposite of highlights. Where highlights add brightness and lighter tones, lowlights blend darker tones. Lowlights are great in hair when a darker but subtle tone is desired. One great way to utilize lowlights is to use them in light or gray hair. Lowlights work like an eraser on light hair and can give the illusion of thicker hair. They can be used to blend out heavy patches of gray and to introduce darker effects without committing to a darker color. In either case, start with just a few streaks and add more if needed.

Baby lights is a term used to describe the micro strand-weaving technique used in highlighting or lowlighting. When baby lights are used in hair coloring, they create a natural effect. They also process well compared to chunkier weaves in the foil packet. When the hair processes in foil, the hair swells from the product and the foil gets warm. Micro strand-weaving processes much faster because the product is saturated within the thin strands in the foil packet. If your strands in the foil are chunky in density, they will process at a much slower speed, especially if not saturated.

Using the panel or slicing technique in highlighting gives a much bolder effect. How you position and strategically place this effect can give a very dramatic highlight. This effect is great for double-process blonding. The panels help to bump up blonding and to give the illusion of multiple tones. This technique is great for lowlighting as well. You can replace dimension and contrast by adding a bold panel where you would like to break the effect up. Even if you're creating bold or thick color lines, it is best to slice or panel thin and repeat the next section immediately adjacent to the first one.

Using foil paper, place it underneath strands and paint on color or lightener. You must place the foil exactly where you want the color to start. So if you're high- lighting from the root, you must bring foil to the scalp. A board can be used to achieve maximum closeness. A highlighting board is a stiff, rectangular board, similar in size to classic white envelopes used for letters or bills. You weave or slice your section, then fold a half-inch of the foil over the board and place it tightly against the root. This makes application a breeze and ensures a close-to-scalp effect. You can also get close by folding the foil over your weaving comb. I personally prefer the board; it gives a sturdy, flat surface on which to apply your color or lightener.

Foil paper is used in applying your formula and securing the formula to maintain the effect. If not for foils or cotton, these effects would be impossible. Traditionally, highlighting or frosting was achieved by using a tight head cap, where a crochet needle would pull strands through perforated holes on the cap. Highlighting caps are still used today on very short hair or fine thin hair, as long as the crochet is consistent, and the holes are tight. When pulling thick hair through the holes, it makes the holes larger, which makes the product susceptible to leaking into the scalp, creating leopard spots, which are a pain to repair. Highlighting caps are not worth it on longer, thicker hair.

In the next chapter, we will differentiate between balayage and ombre and explaining the different meanings and effects produced.

CHAPTER 18

Balayage vs. Ombre

Balayage is a French word meaning to sweep or paint. The technique made its debut in the 1970s in Paris, France. "*Balayage à coton*," as it was originally called, means to strategically sweep color or lightener onto strips of cotton to create a sun-kissed look. How the colorist places the product can determine results from subtle to drastic. This technique allows for a less-uniformed look on the hair, resulting in a natural flow of color. There is no such thing as a blonde balayage or a red balayage. Balayage is not a color; it is a technique.

An ombre color is when the color appears lighter or darker on a horizontal pattern. Ombres typically have a lengthy root with gradually lighter ends, resulting in a gradient of shades.

Following the rules of color theory, ombre effects when done right, can be very drastic and still have a great flow.

Both techniques require little to no maintenance and look better as natural hair grows out. It is popular amongst clients since frequent visits are not needed. Balayage and ombre work best when gradual lightening is done, especially if the client doesn't want their hair cut. Creating this effect in one or two visits requires a lot of time and a lot of skill. Blonde ones are very hard to do on dark hair. However, several different sweeps of color every visit usually makes an amazing ombre. The longer the roots get, the more eye-catching it looks.

The point of these effects is for the color to grow out and to look more sun-kissed and gradient, over time it will look more and more natural. This color effect works great on everyone as long as you follow natural highlights and stick to tones that complement the skin. The effect itself will look great for months. It is currently the most-requested hair trend. If hair coloring is where you want to plant your seeds, you should think about apprenticing at a salon that specializes in hair color. Take many workshops or mentor under a great colorist.

Try new product companies and don't be afraid to experiment. You will find that some clients are eager to try something new. Let the creative juices flow.

This concludes the section on all things color related. Next, we will move on to the section about tools and products. First up is blow drying.

Section 3

All Things Styling

CHAPTER 19

Blow drying

The blow out is a popular service for clients when they want to make their hair instantly look its best. If you blow dry a client's hair well, they will certainly want you to try new services on them. A good blow out gives a great first impression. Knowing how to manipulate someone's hair is a sign that the stylist knows what they are doing. The art of blow drying is a skill of its own.

Blow drying curly hair straight is different than drying naturally straight hair. When drying curly hair to straight, you want it more wet to be able to stretch and pull on the brush and move the blower up and down the shaft until it's dry. The more heat added, the straighter and shinier it will be. Keep the blower moving while you dry to avoid any heat discomfort for your client. Blow drying in even sections will result in a smooth, shiny look.

Straight hair should be whip dried first to remove excess water and moisture. Whip drying is when you shake all the water off and use your fingers to lift and shape the hair. Sometimes whip drying can be used solely to create a tousled, care-free look. I always recommend whip drying 60 percent to cut time and help protect from too much heat damage. It will also give the hair body before you start to blow dry. Straight hair textures just need more body and shape so very wet hair is not recommended.

When blow drying, it's crucial to use the nozzle provided with your dryer to concentrate air flow and avoid scorching the hair. I have counseled many clients who didn't like using the nozzle, thinking it would work quicker without it, who then wondered why their hair burned off. You see, the metal grill on the blower gets very hot and when you press hair against the blower without the nozzle attachment, it can leave grill burn marks or worse break the hair off altogether.

Although I prefer curly locks to dry naturally, a diffuser can be used to speed up the drying time on natural curls. A diffuser is an attachment piece that has a filter to buffer the speed of the dryer and to help avoid any frizzing while drying. Diffusers are quite simple to use, all you do is scrunch the curls repeatedly until the desired drying is achieved.

In the next chapter, we will move onto heat tools and flat irons and whether or not they are needed after the blow dry.

CHAPTER 20

Flat Irons

Heat tools are used to shape hair after a blow dry. You can straighten or curl hair easily and alter it into many shapes. Some hair types need an extra heat tool, either to polish a straight look or to give a curl bouncy movement. These tools are popular; so popular in fact, that most people in the world own heat tools. In a world where we're used to getting things fast, these tools provide the instant gratification we seek.

Flat irons are the number one heat tool most people have. They now come in several different plate sizes. My favorite flat iron is the one-inch Nano titanium by *BaByliss* Pro. The Nano titanium iron technology is amazing; it has a temperature control all the way up to 450 degrees Fahrenheit. It can smooth out coarse hair and tight curly hair like silk. It can also gently smooth out fragile or chemically altered strands by just reducing the heat to a much lower setting.

It is always best to handle chemically and color-treated hair with a gentler heat setting. If more heat is needed, the adjustment can always be made. But if too much heat is used, there's no taking it back.

Bigger flat iron plates do not necessarily mean a faster straightening time. It's just a matter of preference. These bigger plates can create bigger, tousled curls by immediately rotating the strand 180 degrees and then sliding down. This motion is tricky to master; I recommend using a gentler heat setting when practicing.

As opposed to bigger plates, the one-inch flat iron is much better at details and getting close to the scalp. Using the 180-degree rotation mentioned above, it can provide tight, long-lasting curls. How you position the strand on the iron will determine the look of the curl. If you slant the iron, the curls will look dropped and loose. This method curls and waves the hair in a non-conforming way.

In the next chapter, we will discuss wands and other curling irons and when used how they can create their own different types of looks.

CHAPTER 21

Curling Irons & Wands

Curling irons have been around for decades and are still the fastest styling option for curling hair. Whether you use a marcel or a spring iron, you can create a gorgeous array of curls, depending on the size of your irons. As a professional, I prefer to use a marcel iron for its more professional appearance.

A wand is just the rod with a handle, it requires you to manually wrap each section. It is the most client-friendly. It's easy to use and nearly foolproof. All you do is wrap from top to bottom and repeat. Like curling irons, wands come in different sizes to create larger or tighter curls. I tend to use the smaller ones for extra-long hair, heavy hair, or one-length long hair so that the curls will last. If you use too big of an iron, the style can droop fairly quickly.

Layered hair is usually more flattering when curled with a bigger barrel, and it will hold up better due to its different lengths. When curling lobs, bobs, or shorter hair, it is best to work mostly in the center of the shaft to avoid tight and shorter curls unless you're looking for that specific look.

Professional stylists should always have different sizes of irons so that they are prepared to create many different types of looks.

The great thing about heat-styling hair is that the hairstyle can last for a few days. Most clients love to have their hair heat-styled for convenience and to prolong the look. If your clients choose to always heat style, make sure they are getting regular conditioning treatments and trims to prevent the hair from becoming too dry.

Now we can switch gears from heat tools to products. In the following chapters, I will guide you through products stylists must understand so they can be best incorporated into blow drying and heat styling.

CHAPTER 22

Mousse

Products give hair a sense of touch and smell. Clients love the smell of great products and especially love the feel of their favorites. Styling products are to hair what spices are to cooking food: they add a certain flavor to it. Additionally, as a stylist, products aid you in creating long-lasting looks and keeping strands in optimum shape.

Mousse is a foam product added to clean, wet hair. Mousses can be lightweight in the hold to a firmer strength. It is a great base for blowouts to create added volume and perfect for wet-setting rollers for touchable hold. Mousse is also really good on wavy and curly textures if a soft, moist look is desired.

Although firmer mousses exist, too much touching of the hair will diffuse the product and loosen its firmness. Using medium-holding mousse for setting will give the hair a superb shine and help keep the body intact. A heavier mousse would be too stiff and might feel sticky and rough.

Mousse works best on men with fine hair. After a cut and dry, I will foam up a bit of mousse and apply it through the hair. The gentle hold provides just enough product and won't weigh hair down or make it look too wet. I use mousse regularly. One of my specialties is in making fine hair look voluminous and thick, and this product works wonders. The brand name doesn't make too much of a difference aside from scents, but the strength in hold does, so choose wisely.

Mousse has the softest touch and has its uses and strengths. When more hold is needed than mousse alone can provide, it may be mixed with some gel to create this hold or tame thicker strands.

In the next chapter, we will discuss gels, a stiffer medium for styling.

CHAPTER 23

Gels

Gels are a great medium to have on hand when doing hair. They are perfect for applying to wet, thick, curly hair and getting defined strands. When the right hold is needed, gels provide a great pairing to specific curls and slicked-back looks.

Gels are liquid gelatin that helps mold and shape wet hair into a variety of styles. It's great for spiking, wet looks, and firm sets. Gels come in natural hold to extreme hold. Keep in mind, the firmer the gel, the more alcohol in the product. Too much alcohol content can lead to very dry strands.

When gel is applied to curly and wet hair, the hair dries in a perfect curl shape. It may look wet, but it will be dry and stiff to the touch. Gel can be used for slick ponytails too, keeping all stray hairs in place, leaving it wet and shiny-looking. Gel is perfect for thick hair, but not for thin hair, as it will make thin hair look skimpy and much thinner where you see the scalp and the separation from brush or comb strokes.

Spray gels, in my opinion, are the love-child of mousse and gel. They can work great depending on their strength. Use spray gels on wet hair for beachy tousled texture and when setting hair for those retro styles.

In the next chapter, we talk about all moisture products and styling hair with waxes and products for different holding effects.

CHAPTER 24

Wax, Pomade, Clay, Putty, Styling Paste and Volume powder

The following products bring out texture and definition in a cut when applied to dry hair. Using styling paste on a short, choppy pixie haircut makes it look undone and cool. Wax, pomade, clay, putty, and styling paste can all be used for chunking, slicking, taming, defrizzing, and molding. They can range from shiny to matte in finish and can have a variety of hold levels, from soft to strong.

What these products have in common is how they work best on dry hair. For example, say you finished a man's haircut. After you blow- dried and shaped the style, you can add wax to define the shape and give it shine. Wax is a good alternative to gel or mousse, giving hair a more rugged appearance that keeps it thick-looking.

Pomades and styling paste are softer with more shine. Use them to chunk out pieces and separate locks. You can use them to define curls and tame frizz as well. These products are great for drier textures. They help keep the hair moist and can protect it when defining curls with heat tools. Too much of these products on the hair can result in over- saturation. If so, you may need to rewash and start all over. With that in mind, this is a product that does best a bit at a time.

Clays and putties are thicker and concentrated. These are the most matte-finished and tend to be stiff if too much product is used. When applying these, make sure you emulsify the product in your palm to avoid any thick clumping of product in any area, especially in the top sections. While I'm not a big fan of these heavy products, they do work well on certain textures and it never hurts to have multiple products and strengths on hand.

Volume dry powder is also a great product to achieve lift or to tease fine hair. This powder soaks up any moisture where applied and gives quite a lift. Soft, sprinkled-on sections create the best results on most hair. It creates long-lasting volume and adds density and grip to amplify your style.

Now that we have discussed products that work well on dry hair, in the next chapter we will detail what products put in the hair before it dries.

CHAPTER 25

Leave-in Conditioners and Serums

In this chapter, you will learn about the wettest of styling products, ones that work best for moisture-deprived hair. Leave-in conditioners and serums are great products for when optimum moisturizing is needed. Whether dealing with dry hair texture, frizzy curls, or lifeless locks, these products will improve dry to severely dry hair. The specific hair type will determine the level of moisture needed.

Leave-in conditioner is self-explanatory. It's a conditioner that you can leave on. Some, but not all conditioners are very heavy and can leave a film or residue due to its concentration. Leave-in conditioner is a specially formulated more diluted version of conditioner, with the addition of other products that make the leave-in conditioner wearable. The best clients for leave-in conditioner are those with frizzy texture. The leave-in conditioner puts on a coating and helps to tame the hair, creating a soft base for heat styling or for wet locks with mousse or gel on top of it.

Leave-in conditioner also works great as a heat protector for colored hair, applying it on strands before fun-in-the-sun activities like going to a swimming pool or the beach. They are also useful from time to time on most hair, though they are not recommended for greasy hair textures.

Serums are essential for silky-looking hair. They usually smell amazing and can be applied to either wet or dry hair. Serums also create a shiny base for wearing waxes and mousses for defined curls. Some of the serums on the market have silicones, which create a barrier when blow-drying and make curly hair into humidity-free luscious locks. Other serums have things like Moroccan oil, argon oil, olive oil, and castor oil. While these are natural, they are blended with other polymers to create a balance of oil, fragrance, and benzyl salicylate. You can choose between either an all-natural or silicone serums, depending on the client preference and hair type.

In the next chapter, this is the last of the hair product section, we will finish off with hairspray.

CHAPTER 26

Hairspray

Hairspray is my all-time favorite product. When designing hairstyles and creating curls, hairspray gives hair the hold it needs. Hairspray is an aerosol mist produced by a polymer, a solvent, and a propellant. It comes in a soft, touchable hold; flexible hold; medium hold; stronghold; and up to extreme and ultimate hold.

Hairspray is a must for fine hair and a great choice of base to use with heat tools. When using curling irons, adding a soft or flexible hold to the strand before curling can aid in not only the hold but in creating a shiny, neat curl. **Never** use a strong-hold hairspray to curl. Doing so can make the hair stick to the iron and make it unmanageable. Instead, if a stronghold is desired, wait to spray after the curls are finished.

A great way to use soft-flexible hairspray is to calm down flyaways. With most hair, after a blowout, I like to use hairspray to tame flyaways and static down. The static is a natural reaction to having no moisture in the hair. Although I can use waxes or pomades to calm them down, I find that hairspray helps to prolong a style and a blowout. Hairspray is especially needed for creating long-lasting, swept-up looks; for setting a tease for height; and for creating a natural hold without needing any pins. The right hairspray can prolong the life of your blowout, maintaining the body and bounce.

Hairspray can also be in the form of a spritz. Spritz spray can be stiffer, even if a touchable hold is used. When dispensed, it creates a splash of hold all at once. Spritzes are good when stiffer wet looks are desired. Whether you want to lock in a style or spike up a look, just know that spritzes tend to look more wet than aerosol and can be too stiff even with a soft hold because of its splashes when applied. Spritzes are a great choice for creating a shiny, tight-looking ponytail, and they're preferred by ballroom dancers and cheerleaders since they make their hair stay in place while performing.

One of my favorite things to do with hair involves augmenting with hair pieces. In the next chapter, I will explain wigs and hairpieces and different extension methods.

CHAPTER 27

Wigs, Weaves, and Extensions

Wigs, Weaves, and Extensions are still the top leaders in the industry. The WWE business has revolutionized our culture more than ever before. Wigs, in general, have become one of the most sought-after looks. They are so realistic and flattering that some women prefer to only use a wig.

What was once used as a prosthetic for cancer patients, those with thyroid disease, or to cover alopecia spots on the head has become a trend, even over healthy long hair. Everyone, men and women want hair, and the newest technologies in hair replacement are more popular than ever because of the quality and impermanence that comes with them.

Wigs come in many versions, including partials that cover three-quarters of the head and falls, which are flat, square-to-rectangle shaped wig pieces. Most popular in the 1960s, they can usually be used with your hair to make updos and ponytails or used as a short bob to hide long lengths.

Weaves are a fantastic way to have a more permanent hair system. For weaves, the head of the hair is prepared in a braided or netting pattern that the hair wefts will be woven onto. Permanent until removed. They're most commonly used for the client who wants to wear a protective style while they nurse their own hair back to health, or perhaps a client who travels for work and needs to be able to maintain their hair while away. Weaves are the most undetectable and versatile extension method.

Extensions can be added to braided styles as well, from various-sized box braids to full cornrow styles. The styles that have been created by some specialists are remarkable. When having the perfect texture and color to match, a weave can look so realistic that even hair stylists get fooled.

Closures are another popular system to add to wigs and weaves as well. A few inches wide and in an array of lengths, they can be used to create a realistic part in the hair. You can change your color and detail your weave seamlessly. Closures mimic hair and scalp and when blended with makeup they are truly undetectable.

Wefts are perfectly tied strands of hair sewn close together like fringe. Wefts are what get sewn onto wigs and weaves. Technology has even created tape on wefts so they can be instantly applied. Wefts also come in clip-on extensions, made to size. The clip in wefts gives the quickest, safest alternative to augmenting strands. I love working with clip-on hair extensions; they make hair dreams a reality. They thicken a look adding length and volume and giving dark hair color instant color pizazz. Clip-on hair is certainly the ultimate accessory, with the power to transform a look, blending naturally with a client's hair but with temporary ease. Clip-ons are commonly used by clients who like to switch up their more frequently, sometimes even daily. Some clients also like to use extensions as part of a special occasion.

The WWE aspect of the hair industry is surely going to keep rising. With new technologies and products, it is sure to maintain its longevity in hair design.

We have now covered all the things associated with hairstyling, products, tools, and techniques.

From here on out we move into the last part of this book and will focus on customer service and personal development.

Section 4

Building a Professional Mindset

CHAPTER 28

Body language

Aside from a hairstylist paying attention to his or her posture and the positioning of arm movements, the body language I want to address is that of your client. After a great consultation, it is common for your client to feel calm and start to small talk, laugh, and feel trusting. It is up to you to read their body language. If at any time you feel like they have retracted, you must open up communication to see if the client has had a change of heart. You never want to execute a new style until you know their body language feels right.

I have a love of ultra-long hair, so when cutting drastically or changing to a whole different look, I express that the look will be drastic, and that I want to ensure the client feels extremely comfortable and confident that they want to cut short. There are times when you will be asked for your opinion, it can be nerve-wracking but exciting. If a client is really enthusiastic about the cut, continue the discussion cutting little by little and talking with them throughout the process to help guide them through the amazing creation. This will make the effort very gratifying.

I've come to appreciate assertive and blunt clients as well, for they tell you what they want and what they don't want right away. This is excellent because now you will suggest something within their guidelines and discuss how to proceed. Sometimes it's the smallest change, but the client feels at ease because they trust you. I also think quiet clients are great because they let me focus and allow my creative juices to start flowing quicker. It's the unsure clients that cause the most work. This is a client who shows you a new look they want to try out but has doubts and wants you to convince them. Everyone has a different perception of subtle to drastic, so it's best to make very limited choices for the client to decide within.

Learning how to read a client's body language is crucial, especially if you perceive an ounce of doubt.

My next chapter is just about how to be completely honest and knowing when to admit what you can and can't do.

CHAPTER 29

Be Honest

Let's face it. We can't please everyone! This is something I learned not too long ago. Sometimes things are far beyond what you can do and guarantee. People actually respected me more as a professional when I sent them to a different stylist who can execute what they are looking for. Within the field of hair design, some of us are cutters, some are colorists, some are barbers, some are wig designers and chemical specialists. It's great to know other specialists so you can give the right referrals. We all have special talents and we all love to work in what we specialize in.

If you have a referral for a great colorist, mention it. If you know of a fantastic barber, tell your client. You don't have to know everything; you can create a great business by simply specializing in what you do best. You will work more comfortably knowing you can guarantee a job well done. I specialize mostly in haircutting, hairstyling, updos, extensions, and wigs. I love to drastically change someone who is daring. The excitement and eagerness I feel from a client really makes my cutting come to life.

The style is the choice of the wearer. So what if you have a long face or a square face. A client shouldn't have to limit themselves to what society or style claims they should be. I would rather see someone wear a short, confident cut rather than hide behind long hair because of their weight. Or find a way to switch up a style for someone who hides a long forehead behind bangs. I love to offer people choices and ideas.

When I do extensions or create a wig or hairpiece for a client, this gives me joy as well, especially if someone does not have the length they desired or if a client has lost their hair due to medications or medical conditions and treatments like chemotherapy. It always puts a smile on my face knowing I can help with what I love to do and when I can suggest something that they didn't think would be possible.

I remember a client who wanted a slanted, longer-in-the-front style but had short bangs. For those longer, slanted looks, your bangs or front layers must be longer than the back to create the effect. I was able to clip in a couple of extensions in her bang and crown area that matched her hair perfectly, and she was ecstatic. When I suggested the clip-ins, I thought it fit the moment and it so happened that I had a few clips left over from a previous project. I wasn't even going to sell them to her. I wanted to gift her them because I knew she would appreciate it. She ended up ordering a complete set of hair extensions because she was so impressed that I could change her look dramatically. It was the best upsell I never meant to do.

When you truly work from the heart and take pride in what you do, people can see and feel that. Being able to make a cancer patient happy and cry tears of joy because they love their wig is the most gratifying feeling I've known; I made someone smile from my gift. It's a gift I love to share, to be in the moment and enjoy the time of change or excitement in my clients' lives.

All that said, being honest does not mean to talk negatively about else's work. In the next chapter, we'll talk about staying in your lane and never to talk badly about another coworker or stylist.

CHAPTER 30

Never speak ill about another stylist

I have always stayed out of commenting negatively about another stylist's work. Not only does it make you look bad, but it demotes your credibility as a professional.

There is something so intimate and safe about going to a stylist that makes people want to pour out their life stories and share things they probably wouldn't tell their close friends or family. The things I have heard through my experience behind the chair has been mind-blowing. Even things I never wanted to know. Yes, I've had a chit-chat and many laughs, but in the end, the conversation isn't the goal, whether serious or lighthearted. It is your job to do great work and move on to the next client.

As a stylist, I love to hear about a client's hair history and their goals for the future of their hair. I give suggestions and recommendations about what to do next. I believe in creating a great experience for the client and use my platform to educate and execute.

Gossip is something else to avoid while styling. To gossip about other clients and stylists to your clients makes it look like you don't have any regard for your career. Ask yourself what the impression is you are leaving with the client. Will they feel comfortable telling you something vulnerable about their hair? Will they respect you as a professional?

You want to be able to grow in your craft to stand out as a professional and to make potential clients want to seek you out for the impeccable services you provide. If a client goes to you, it should be because you make them feel great with your special techniques and services, they haven't gotten anywhere else. Don't undermine this with what you choose to talk about.

You must remember to strive to be the best hairstylist you can be, one who can take their talents and services to new heights.

A positive outlook on life can help you grow in amazing directions.

In my next chapter, I implore that you get creative and have fun by thinking outside the box.

CHAPTER 31

Creativity and thinking outside the box

You must learn to think outside the box. Eventually, you get used to using the same patterns and techniques. You can probably do many things with your subconscious but imagine how great it would be to channel your creativity to a whole new level and to be able to instantly imagine a new look on your client. This vivid imagination is part of thinking outside the box. You will get an experimental client who will let you create, and you will also have the one who wants exactly what they asked for.

When I look at a hairstyle, I typically imagine what steps I will do first. For instance, if a client shows me a picture of her desired look, whether it's a cut, color, or style, I'm already planning the steps in my head and suggesting possibilities to get the client there with me. At times, I will do something unconventional such as asymmetrical shapes or drastic disconnected looks like a shaved undercut. That's how new trends are created and whole makeover moments experienced. You get excited about what you are about to create and execute a true work of art.

It's important as a professional to experiment and try new things. Sometimes, when I cut someone's hair really short, I create a few shapes in the process to experiment with new ideas or to see if the person may like what I've done so far. I have sometimes changed the look if a client has a change of heart. You can always cut shorter, but you can never put cut hair back on. You must cut in a pattern that allows for creative changes if necessary.

Test different colors on a client who isn't afraid of your suggestions. This is a great opportunity to use a color that maybe not everyone likes or one that is perhaps too red or too drastic for someone. If the client lets you decide, that is the time to think outside the box. These experimental moments make hairdressing exciting, and in these moments the best hair color formulas get created.

As I encourage you to do amazing designs and create bold and fun colors, always remember that no one is too old or too much of an expert to learn. Practice makes perfect, and people who continue to educate themselves truly become masters at their craft.

In the next chapter, we will talk about the importance of education and how it's important to always continue to learn.

CHAPTER 32

Always continue to learn

The most successful hairstylists always remain humble and continue to learn. Just because someone makes tons of money or works on the most prestigious clients does not mean you have made it—unless that is all you desire. Learning a new technique or a new way of doing something feeds your brain and expands your creativity. Many times I have encountered stylists with huge egos, who won't share ideas or teach someone who loves to learn out of fear that a student would surpass them or even take their clients away.

I find it flattering when a fellow stylist asks if I can show them how to do what I do. If I teach someone how to do something and they master it, it is the utmost compliment. Maybe it's because I love what I do or because I love to learn and teach alike. Doctors, dentists, mechanics, and many other professionals all continue their education. Continuing education leads us to a better understanding of new technology and current trends.

The hair industry is constantly changing and evolving. There are always new techniques to learn and new products launching. Education is also a great way to expand our experience and perhaps find new alternatives. Of course, we all have those go-to products and tools that give us the results we need, so we find it hard to break the pattern and try something new. I'm guilty of this as well, but I've also found myself pleasantly surprised when I did try something new.

I remember I was once addicted to a specific serum. It was the right amount of oil and moisture and had such a great fragrance to it. I loved using it right after a blow dry and swore I would never use any other serum. One day, I was out of it and quickly went to the supply store to pick up a bottle. I was shocked to hear they didn't carry that brand anymore and I was forced to try something new. Although I was reluctant at first, the store clerk assured me I would love this alternative, and boy was she right. She listened to what I loved about the previous product and gave me an even better suggestion. If I hadn't run out of the serum and been forced to try a new one, I would have never known that I would love this new suggestion even more. The fragrance was heaven and the product was so great and concentrated that I didn't even need to use as much.

Our industry is saturated with education, workshops, and inspiration. There are mentors, coaches, and educators for these specific outlets. Never stop learning, despite your status, age, or ego. There is always something that could change how you see the beautiful world of hairstyling. You might be surprised at what you will learn.

Take these tips, tricks, tools, and techniques and make them your own. In fact, create some of your own. There are many outlets to choose from in the beauty industry. Find the one that best suits you and truly makes you feel great. Take control of your career and follow your heart.

AUTHOR BIO

Raymond Negron has been a professional and licensed cosmetologist since 1999. Located in New Jersey he provides hair styling, wig making and cutting services for weddings and other special events across the United States and internationally. When I was young, I realized that cutting and styling hair was where my true passion lay. I realized that I have a passion to help people look and feel their best. Since obtaining his cosmetology license Raymond has continued in obtaining additional licenses and certifications in various specialties such as the Structure in Motion and Hair Styling, Temptu Hair Brushing and Mud Make-Up Designer for Beauty and Makeup in Film.

For additional information about Raymond and his products, please visit https://www.hairstylist101.com

Made in the USA
Middletown, DE
16 April 2019